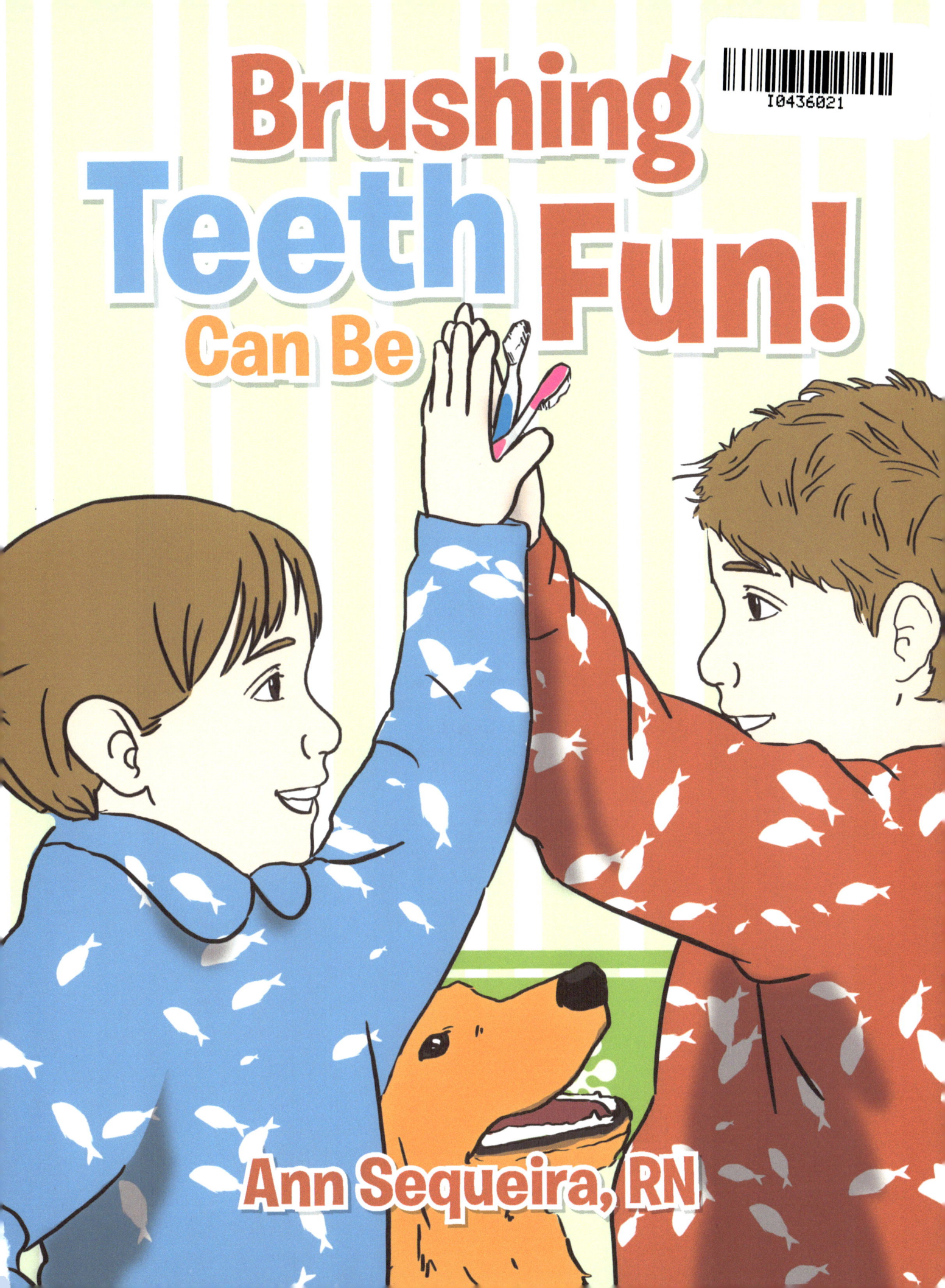

This book is dedicated to my daughter,
Chloe, who inspired me to write this book.

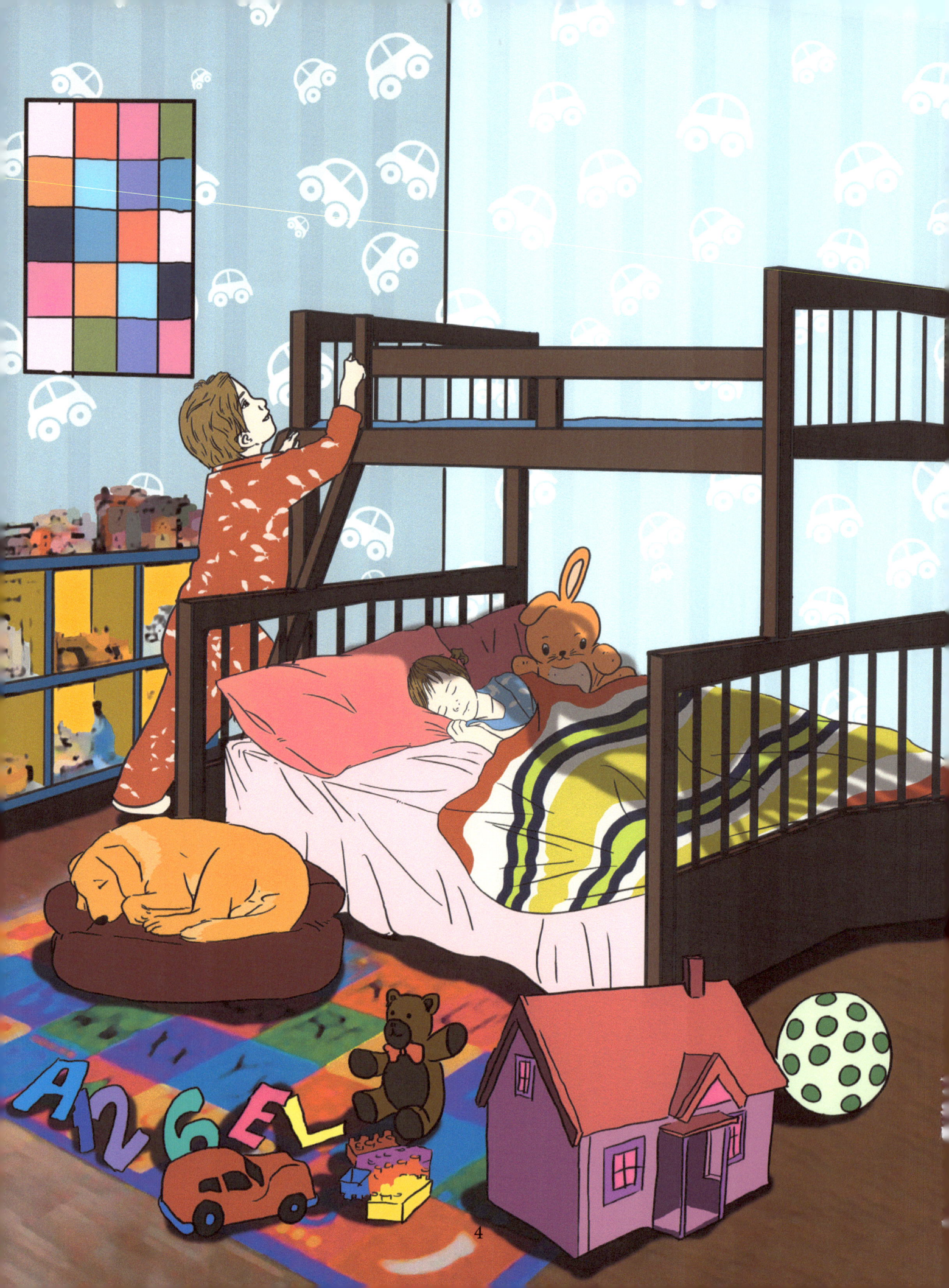

Jack woke up. He climbed down from his bunk bed. He went to the bathroom, and started applying toothpaste to his toothbrush.

His three-year-old sister, Jill, walked in after him. "Jack, what are you doing?" Jill asked.

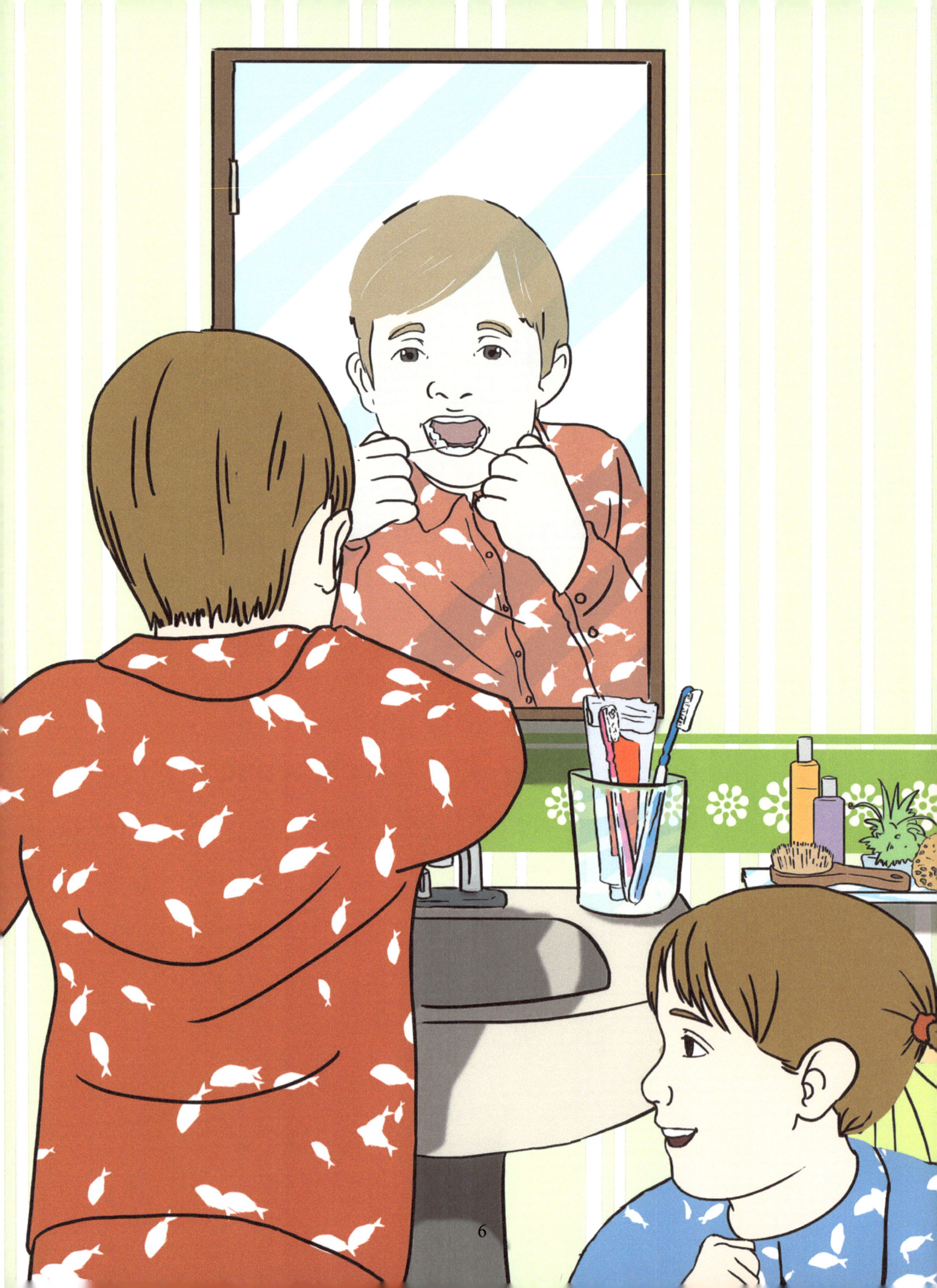

Jack picked up the floss.

Jill pointed to it and asked, "What
is that, Jack? I WANT THAT!"
"This is floss."

Jack handed her the floss.
Jill touched the thread.

He asked, "Would you like to try it?"

Jill held the floss in her hands.

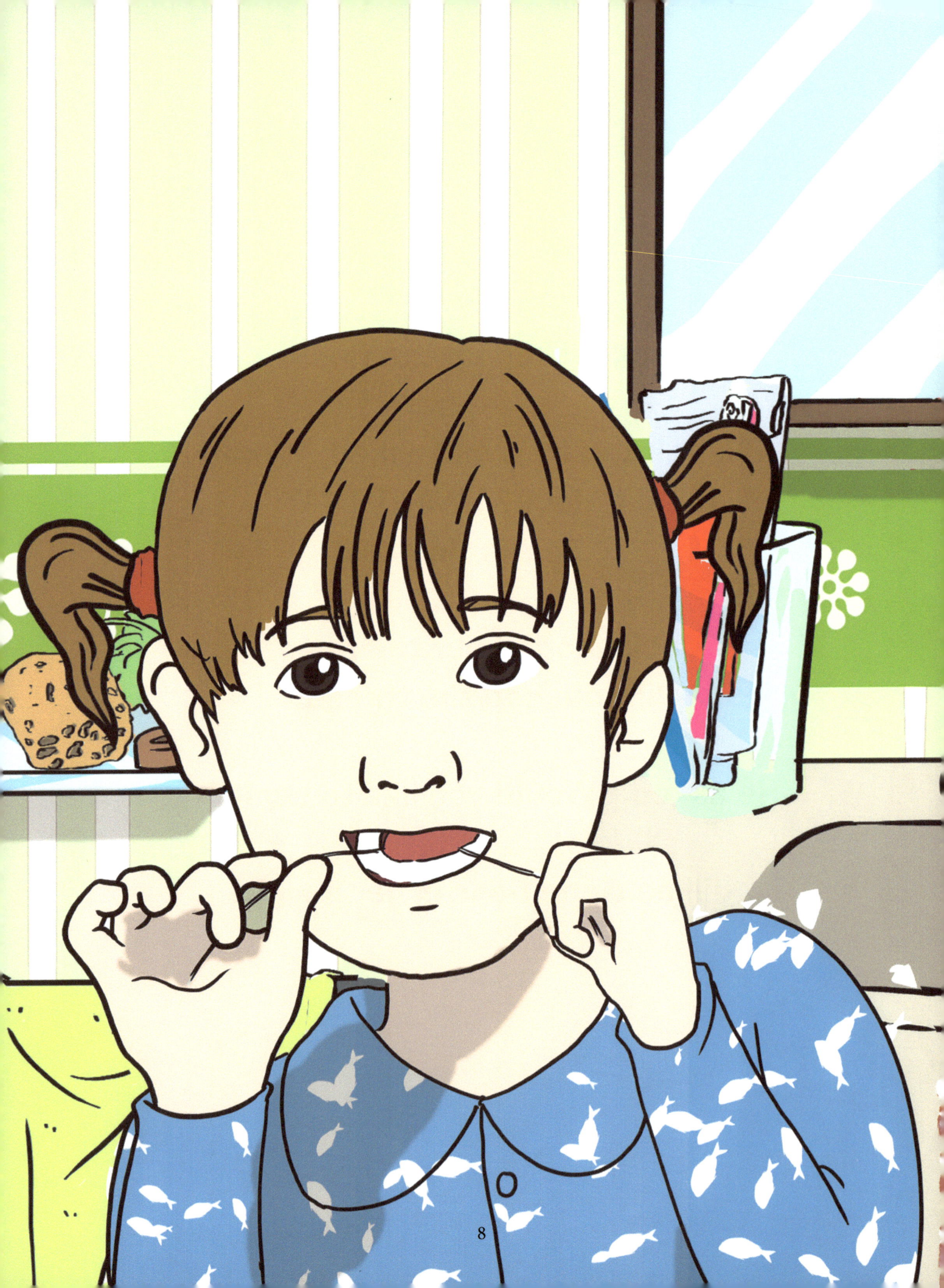

She moved the floss between her teeth, just like Jack. That felt different.

Then Jack started brushing his teeth.

"Jack, what are you doing?" asked Jill.

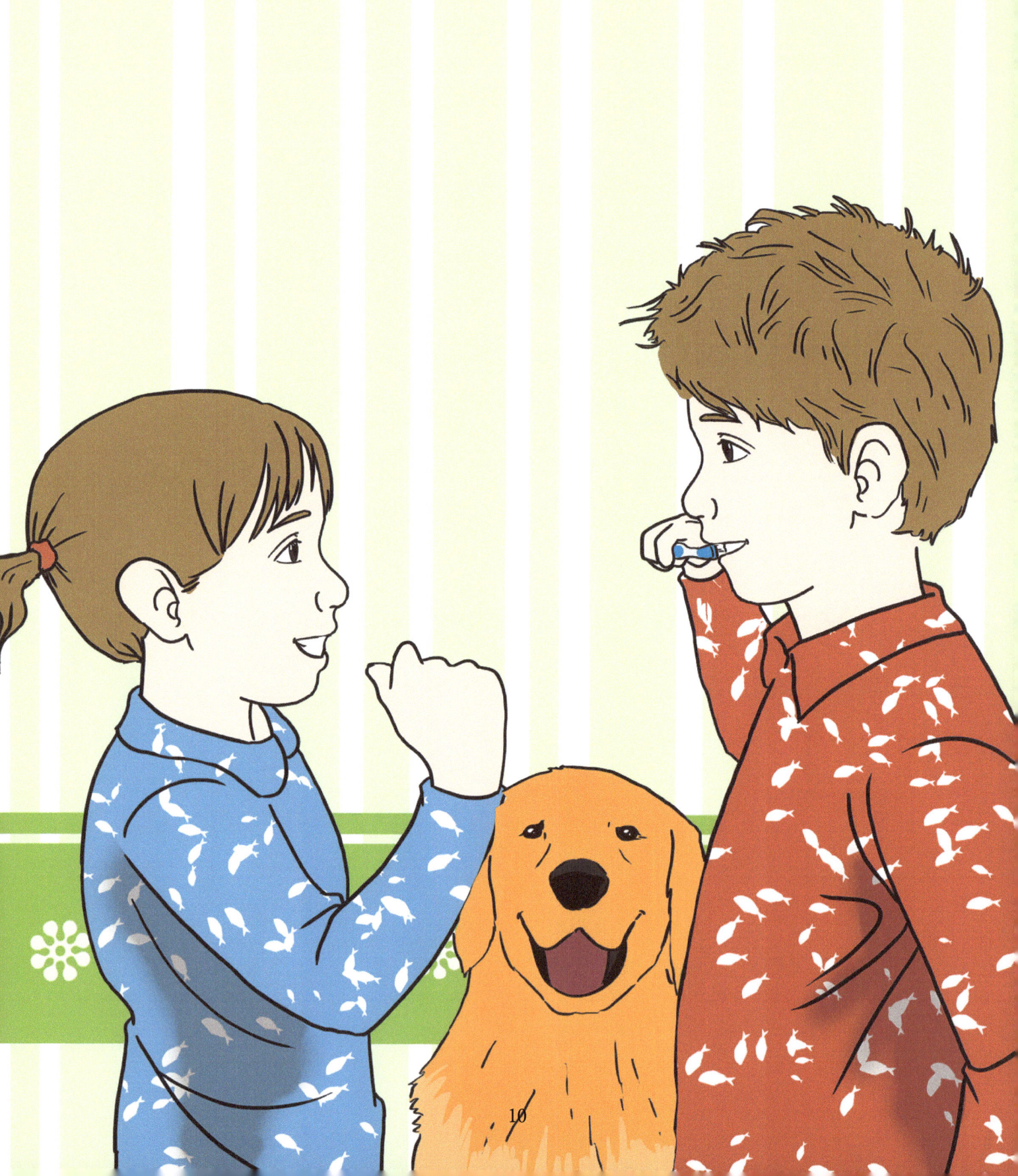

10

"I'm brushing my teeth 'because
we have germs on them."

"You mean we have teeth with germs?"
She giggled.

Jill wanted to do whatever Jack did,
and grabbed her toothbrush.

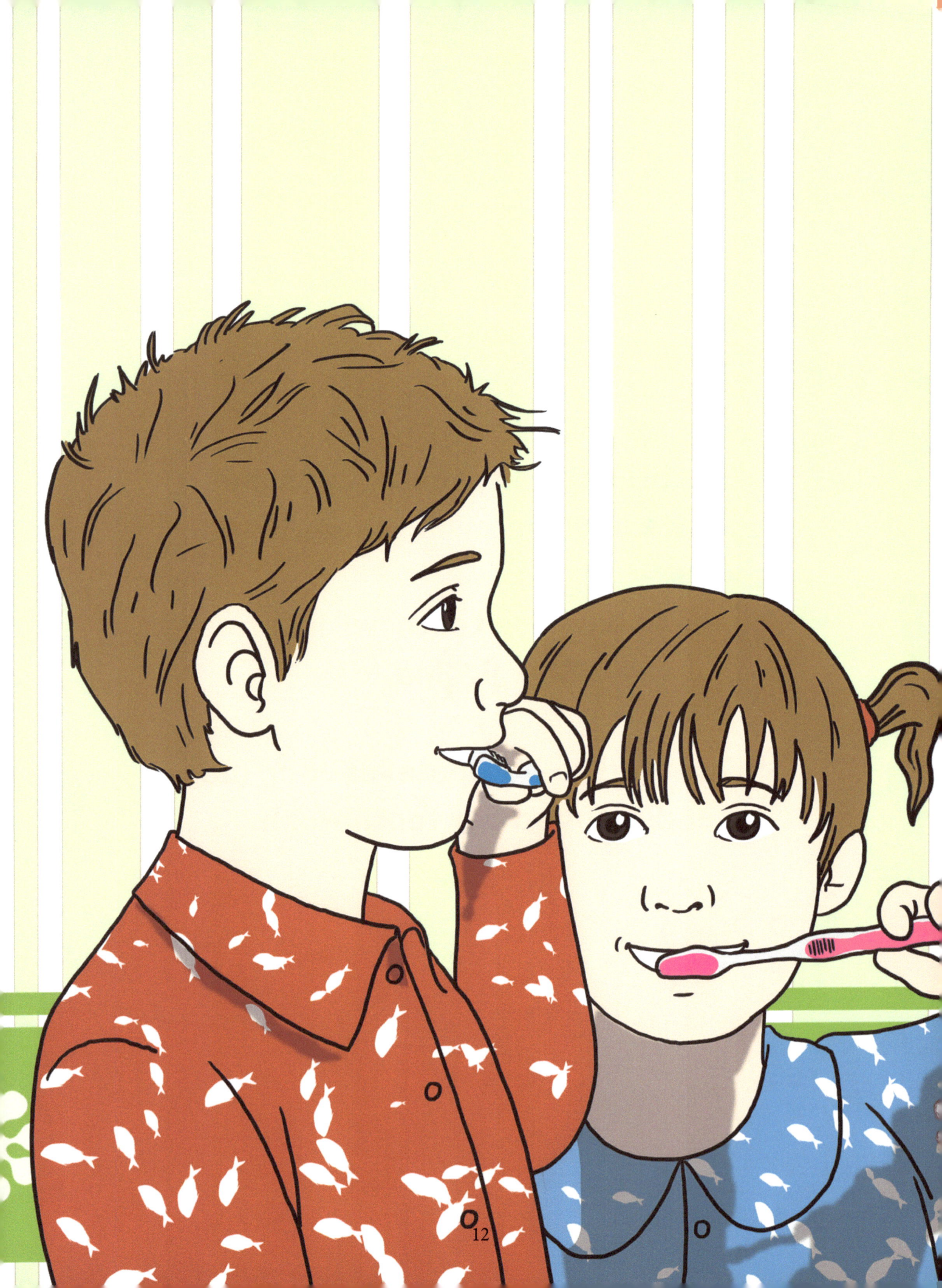

Jack brushed the front of his teeth.

So, Jill brushed the front of her teeth too.

Jack brushed the back of his teeth.

So, Jill tried to do the same.

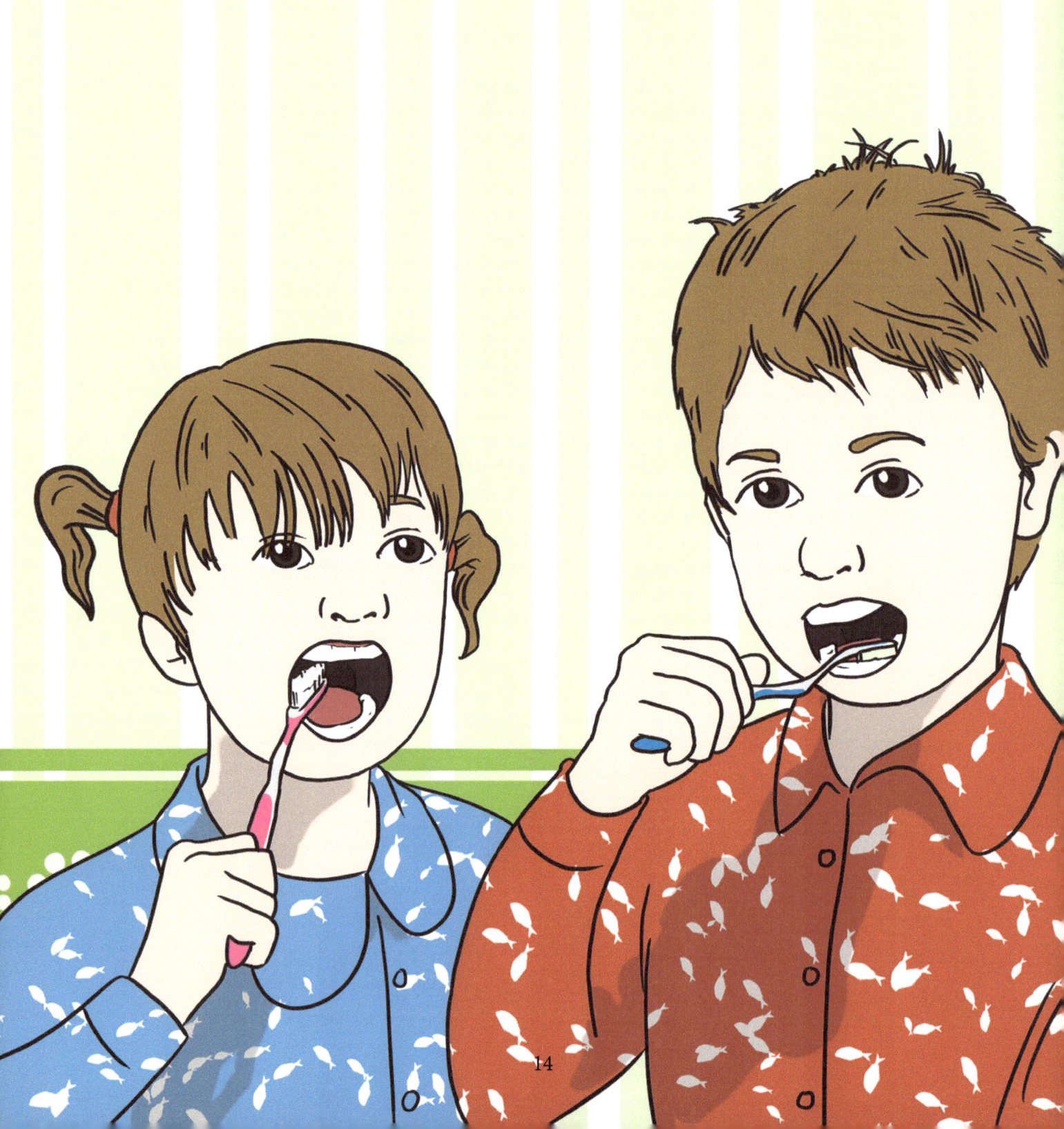

14

Jack brushed the inner sides of his teeth.

Jill hurried to copy him.

Jill moved her brush up and
down, all around.

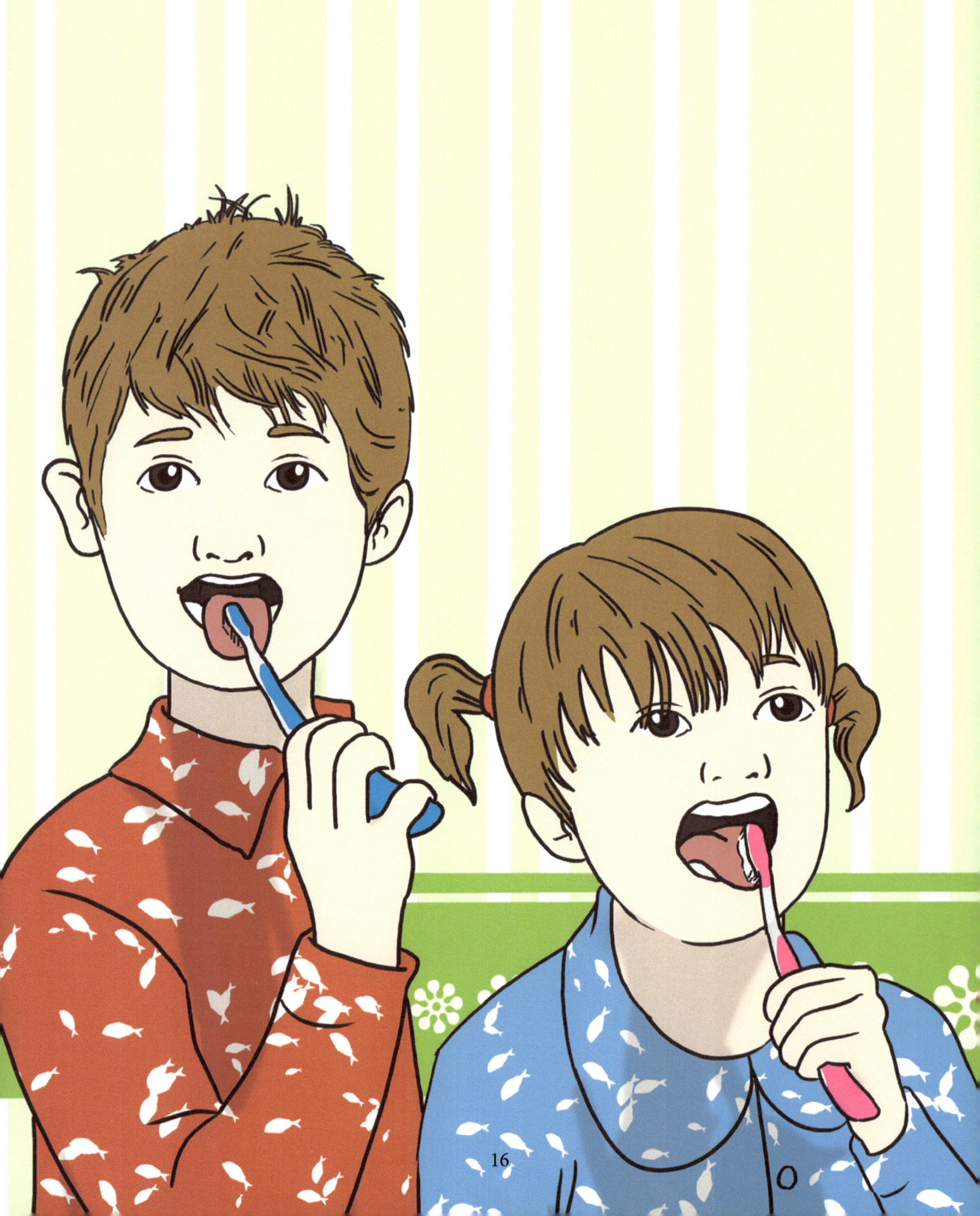

Jack brushed his tongue.

Jill tried to copy her brother.

That felt funny. It tickled. She

looked at Jack. Jack laughed.

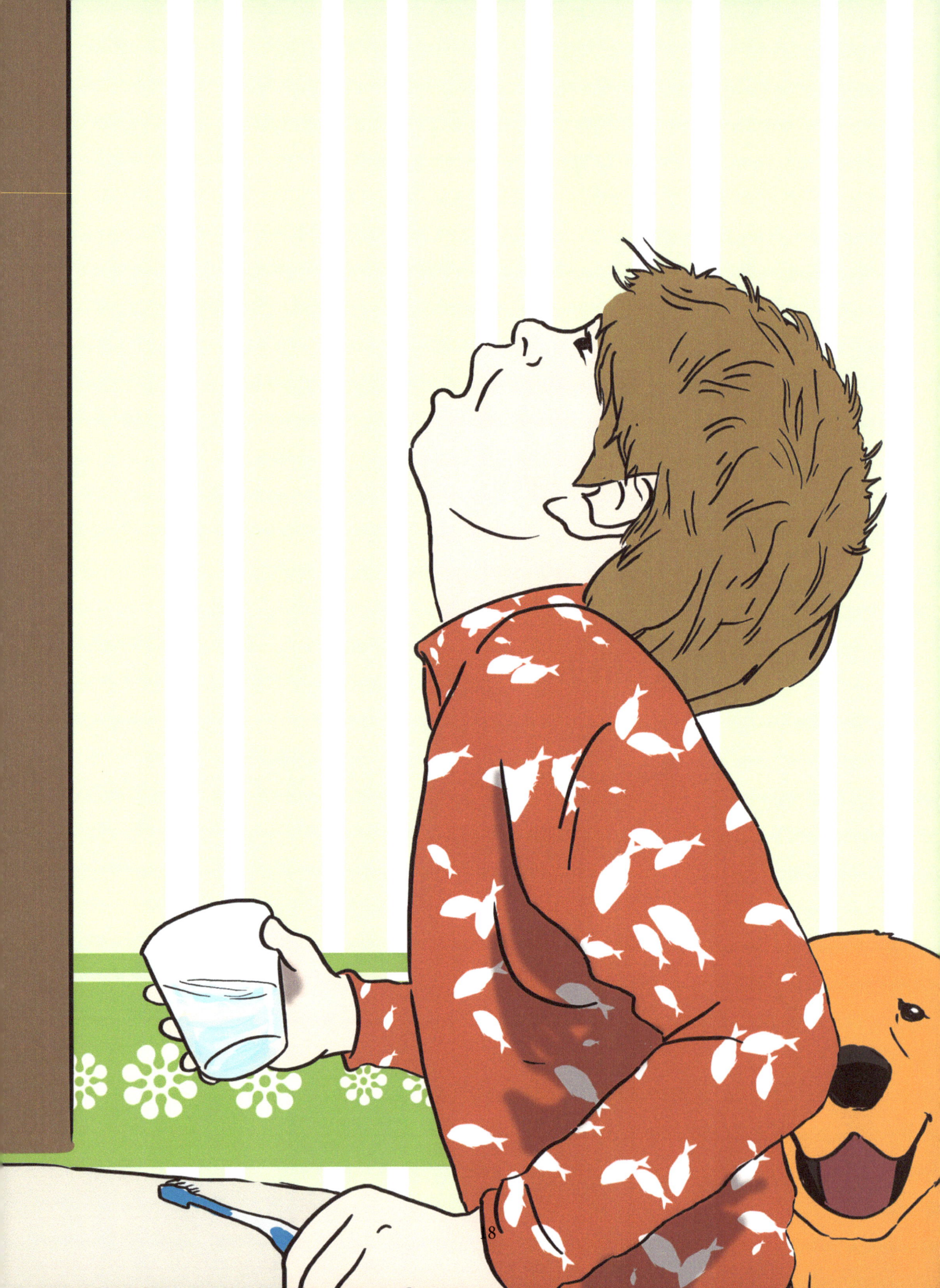

Finally, Jack gargled with the mouthwash.

The gargle made a funny sound,
and Jill laughed.

Jill tried the mouthwash. She tried to gargle on
the sweet blue-coloured water,
but instead of gargling, she swallowed it.

Jack laughed. "Nice try," he said.

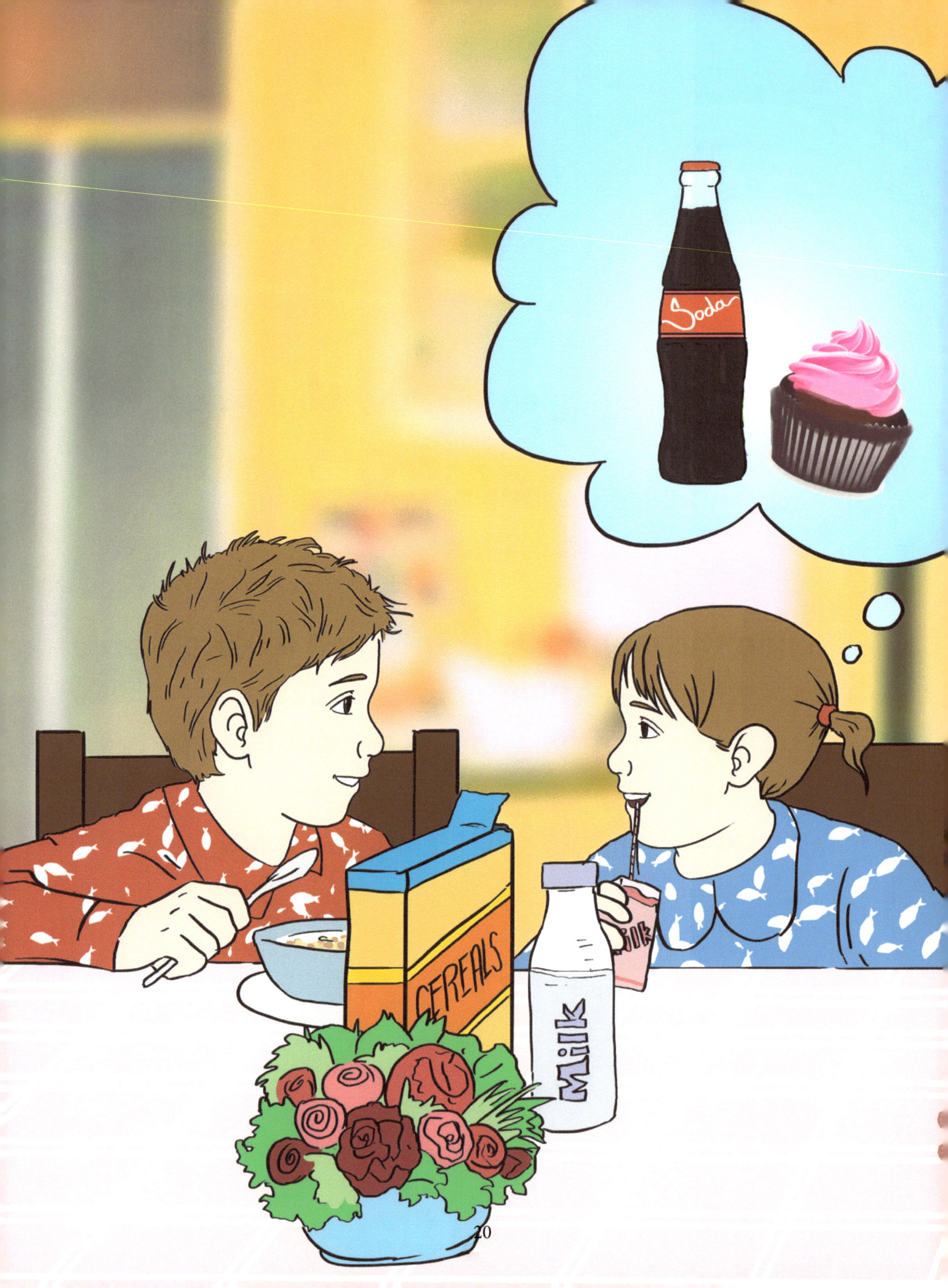

Then Jack went to the breakfast table. Jill quickly followed him.

Jack poured some cereal and milk.

Jill climbed on the seat next to her brother.

"I don't want cereal, I want a cupcake".

Jack laughed. "No, Jill, no cupcakes. They are not good for your teeth."

"But, I want soda. I want candy."

"Yes, I know you do, but you cannot have goodies for breakfast. You can have these sugary treats only sometimes."

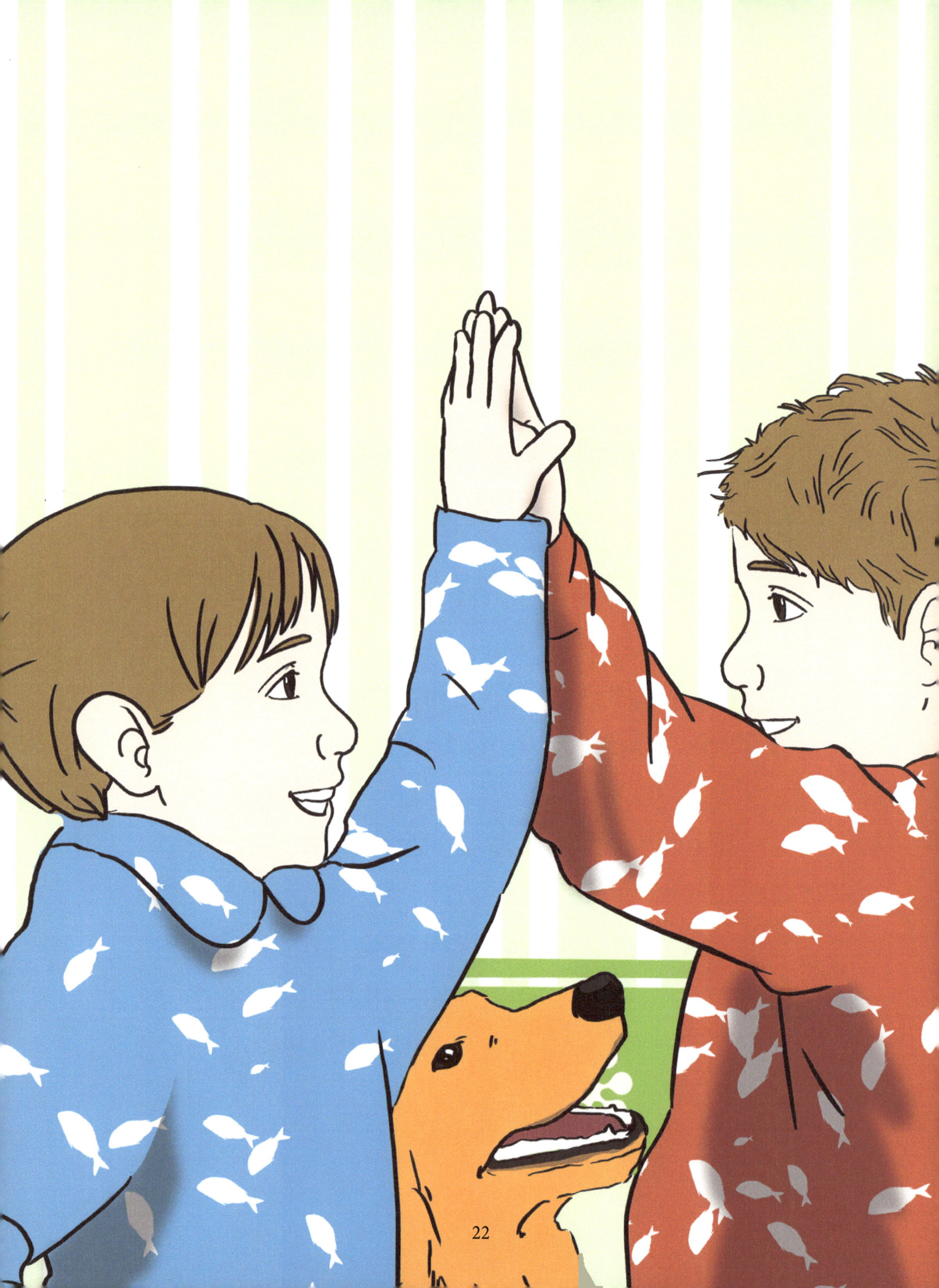

"Okay?" said Jack softly.

"Okay," replied Jill.

Jack handed Jill a cup of milk.

"I know a song, and it goes like this" he sang

FRUITS, FRUITS, EAT YOUR FRUITS.
EAT THEM EVERY DAY.

MERRILY, MERRILY, MERRILY,
HEALTHY TEETH ALL DAY.

VEGGIES, VEGGIES, EAT YOUR VEGGIES.

EAT THEM EVERY DAY.
THEN YOU'LL HAVE A HEALTHY SMILE
AND HAPPY TEETH ALL DAY.

"I like this song," Jill told Jack.

"I know you do," said Jack and, they gave each other a high five.

The End